Summa

G000048778

The Obesity Code

Unlocking the Secrets of Weight Loss

by Jason Fung, MD

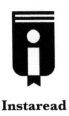

Instaread

Please Note

This is a summary with analysis.

Table of Contents

Overview

The Obesity Code addresses the history, causes, and treatments of obesity and today's rising obesity rates. By understanding it through scientific and social study, obesity becomes less of a blanket term for metabolic complications and a more tangible problem with real, though not widely practiced, solutions.

The main problem with treating obesity is that many doctors and their obese patients don't know what actually causes obesity. Often, health experts believe that weight gain results from consuming too many calories while not expending enough calories, a theory known as "calories in, calories out." However, decades of research has proven that this obesity model is problematic and over-simplified. Calorie consumption and expenditure are not independent of each other. If people decrease calorie consumption in an effort to lose weight, their body compensates by slowing down processes such as metabolism to expend fewer calories. Also, exercise is not nearly as instrumental in weight loss as was once thought, as basal metabolism governs a much larger percentage of energy expenditure. Instead, obesity is the result of a hormonal imbalance primarily caused by insulin levels that spike for too long. Sustained, high insulin levels signal the body to maintain a regular weight that is too high. This makes it difficult to prevent plateauing after short-term weight loss and subsequent weight gain.

Diet is the most important factor in both short-term and long-term weight loss. By eating the right foods at the right times, people can better control their levels of insulin and insulin resistance and better manage their weight over the long term.

Important People

Jason Fung is the author of the book and a physician who specializes in treating kidney diseases. In the process of determining the best practices for treating his patients, he uncovered truths about obesity that have widespread implications for patients suffering from obesity, diabetes, and other metabolic complications.

Key Takeaways

1. The status quo for medical treatment for obesity—decreasing calories in, increasing calories out—doesn't work, yet doctors continue to prescribe it.

2. Exercise does not play as large a role in weight loss and obesity as some experts believe.

3. Obesity occurs when hormones become unbalanced and signal the body to maintain a higher weight.

4. Research has linked obesity to high-glycemic carbohydrates, also known as refined carbohydrates.

5. Sugar intake is a key factor in obesity, and sugar-sweetened drinks are one of the main culprits in weight gain.

6. Fiber has a number of health benefits; it reduces absorption of carbohydrates.

7. To overcome obesity, individuals need to lose weight in the short term and redetermine their body weight set point in the long term by breaking the cycle of insulin resistance.

8. Obesity has multiple causes and therefore requires several different targets and treatments to overcome each individual factor.

Analysis

Key Takeaway 1

The status quo for medical treatment for obesity—decreasing calories in, increasing calories out—doesn't work, yet doctors continue to prescribe it.

Analysis

Sometimes medical treatments become common practice for doctors and common knowledge for patients even in the face of research that suggests they are ineffective or even harmful. One such treatment is the energy balance theory, also known as "calories in, calories out," which claims that people should lose weight if they decrease their intake of calories while increasing their caloric expenditure. However, numerous studies over the past several decades have proved this theory to be false, and the obesity rate has continued to rise in spite of this practice. Still, health care providers and even the

US government stand by this theory as the best way to combat obesity.

According to a 2015 Nielsen survey, 41 percent of global respondents said that eating smaller portions—or in other words, calorie reduction—was their chosen diet strategy. [1] It was more common than any other weight-control strategy. In North America, portion control was even more popular, with nearly half of respondents practicing some form of it. Those percentages demonstrate just how prevalent calorie reduction continues to be as a treatment for obesity. Calorie reduction may have been a recommendation from an individual's doctor. Or dieters may have implemented this strategy on their own, based on inaccurate assumptions about calories that they've heard their whole lives.

This belief system may be starting to shift. More than one-third of Nielsen's respondents, 37 percent, said their tactic was to consume fewer processed foods. In North America, that number was even higher, at 46 percent, the highest of any region. In addition, 57 percent of respondents said they were adding more natural and fresh foods to their diet, an uptick from 55 percent in Nielsen's 2011 survey. These numbers suggest that more people are recognizing the importance of the types of food and beverages they consume rather than just the amount of calories they intake.

Key Takeaway 2

Exercise does not play as large a role in weight loss and obesity as some experts believe.

Analysis

Exercise is only one factor in calorie expenditure. And it's a less important factor relative to basal metabolic rate, which is the energy expended through bodily processes such as maintaining body temperature and liver or kidney function. Theories abound that increased inactivity has led to the rise of obesity, but various studies have debunked those theories. If a lack of exercise does not cause people to gain weight, then increasing exercise isn't likely to help people lose weight either.

A study published in February 2016 suggests that more exercise does not necessarily equate to higher levels of energy expenditure. [2] Researchers concluded that instead, people who are exercising more than average eventually reach a plateau. After that plateau, any gains made are relatively insignificant. Moderate exercise did lead to more calories burned than for participants who were sedentary. But once someone worked out beyond the "sweet spot," as researchers called it, calorie expenditure reached a ceiling. [3]

Key Takeaway 3

Obesity occurs when hormones become unbalanced and signal the body to maintain a higher weight.

Analysis

Hormones perform critical functions throughout the body including regulating weight management systems, such as appetite, blood sugar levels, and fat storage. Insulin is a fundamental hormone for fat storage. It regulates the amount of glucose in the bloodstream from any carbohydrates consumed. When insulin levels are too high, fat accumulates around the body. If sustained over time, obesity results.

Many studies have been conducted to examine the relationship of hormones such as leptin and ghrelin, which impact weight regulation, on obesity and weight management. A 2014 study demonstrated a correlation of increased levels of leptin and decreased levels of ghrelin in obese patients with metabolic disorder. [4] These hormonal imbalances appear in addition to the metabolic complications caused by imbalance of the hormone insulin, which illustrates the complexities of hormonal regulation in conjunction with weight management. Other studies have examined the relationship of hormonal imbalances, including ghrelin, leptin, and insulin, with obesity in the context of lifestyle factors such as sleep, stress, and meal timing. [5]

Key Takeaway 4

Research has linked obesity to high-glycemic carbohydrates, also known as refined carbohydrates.

Analysis

Consuming high-glycemic carbohydrates, such as refined white sugar and white flour, leads to spikes in blood sugar. High blood sugar increases insulin levels and high insulin levels have been proven to cause weight gain. Therefore, consuming high-glycemic carbohydrates is thought to cause weight gain. However, that causation is not conclusive based on varied research, and other factors may impact increased insulin levels. Still, experts believe that increased intake of refined carbohydrates played a role in the rising rate of obesity in the United States over the past several decades.

Proponents of low-fat and low-carb diets continue to be at odds today. Both sides can produce research to support their theories. Other studies show no statistically significant difference in weight loss between calorie-restrictive, low-fat diets and low-carb diets. [6] According to Nielsen's 2015 survey, low-fat diets were still much more common than low-carbohydrate, high-fat diets, at 65 percent of respondents versus only 25 percent. [7] North America was slightly below both averages while maintaining the same trend, with 59 percent of North American respondents reducing their fat intake versus 23 percent following a low-carb, high-fat diet.

Following the low-carb dieting trend, common carbohydrate products such as bread and cereal saw sales declines of 3 percent and 8 percent respectively between 2012 and 2014. Developed regions such as North America and Europe drove the trend. Cereal sales have been falling for the past decade after peaking in the mid-1990s. Processed cereal, known to contain sugar and refined carbohydrates, has suffered as breakfast food competitors such as Greek yogurt appeal to health-conscious consumers. [8]

Key Takeaway 5

Sugar intake is a key factor in obesity, and sugar-sweetened drinks are one of the main culprits in weight gain.

Analysis

As reducing dietary fat intake became the focus of weight-loss methods, sugar intake increased significantly. The rise in sugar consumption coincided with the rise of obesity in the United States. Sugar-sweetened drinks have driven this increase in part because it is so easy to consume liquid calories. This includes diet soda, which soda companies have said could be part of a healthy diet. However, the artificial sweeteners used in diet soda have linked diet soda to weight gain.

National and international health organizations have voiced concerns about high sugar intake. In 2015, the World Health Organization recommended a reduction in sugar consumption to 10 percent of daily calorie intake. [9] Over the next year, both the US Food and Drug Administration (FDA) and 2015 US Dietary Guidelines echoed that recommendation. [10] Also in 2015, the FDA proposed a supplemental rule that would update the Nutrition Facts label on food and beverage products to reflect the amount of added sugars they contain. Processed foods, such as condiments and tomato sauce, are notoriously high in added sugars.

State and city governments are stepping in to ameliorate overconsumption of sugar in the United States.

Several are proposing soda taxes, such as the tax passed in Berkeley, California, in 2014. [11] Berkeley was the first city to pass such a tax in the United States. The one-cent-per-ounce excise tax has increased local retail prices for sugary drinks, according to a 2015 study, but findings did not confirm what dietary impacts the tax has had, if any. In 2016, up to a dozen or more US cities could see a sugary-sweetened beverage tax introduced in their local legislature, according to public health advocates. [12]

Although diet soda may not have sugar or calories, the alternative sweeteners it contains bring their own health concerns. A 2010 review of studies on artificial sweeteners concluded that artificial sweeteners may actually contribute to weight gain. [13] The psychological impact of drinking a beverage marketed as diet-friendly may also come into play with other dietary choices. A 2016 review of survey data concluded that diet beverage drinkers may make up for the lack of calories in their drinks by eating other foods with high levels of sugar, sodium, fat, and cholesterol, also known as "discretionary foods." [14]

Key Takeaway 6

Fiber has a number of health benefits; it reduces absorption of carbohydrates.

Analysis

Fiber is non-digestible and is often consumed as part of a carbohydrate. Consuming fiber has many health benefits, though the exact mechanisms aren't entirely understood. For example, fibrous foods need to be chewed more and tend to be denser, which can help reduce intake and increase fullness. Fiber is also an anti-nutrient, which means it can reduce absorption and digestion of nutrients. Most notably, fiber reduces absorption of carbohydrates, which then leads to lower blood glucose and insulin levels. Some cultures maintain high-carbohydrate diets, but those carbohydrates are unprocessed and, therefore, high in fiber. These people can maintain healthier weights than those who follow diets based on processed foods.

When researchers discovered dietary fiber's anti-nutrient capabilities, they first considered it a detrimental characteristic. Cereal manufacturers developed technology in the late nineteenth century to create cereals and flours that were low in or devoid of dietary fiber. [15] Since then, research has proven these anti-nutrient capabilities to be beneficial, such as in the prevention of chronic diseases or the negative effects of carbohydrate absorption.

One subset of dietary fiber that is gaining attention is prebiotics. Prebiotics are fermented ingredients that impact the composition or activity of the bacteria located in the gut. Healthy gut bacteria composition has primarily been associated with improved gut health, which potentially leads to overall health and well-being. Among other foods, including some grains, vegetables such as leeks, garlic, onions, asparagus, chicory, and Jerusalem artichokes are all good sources of prebiotics. Prebiotics' ability to improve gut health has made them a focus of contemporary nutrition research. [16]

Key Takeaway 7

To overcome obesity, individuals need to lose weight in the short term and redetermine their body weight set point in the long term by breaking the cycle of insulin resistance.

Analysis

All diets can both succeed and fail when it comes to losing weight. After a certain amount of time, anyone following any particular diet runs the risk of plateauing and eventually regaining weight. After losing a certain amount of weight, the body reacts by prompting changes in bodily processes to encourage weight gain until the body is back to its original body weight set point. The body weight set point is the weight level at which the body naturally gravitates back to if weight is gained or lost beyond that point. If people try to continue to lose weight, they could be working against their own brain. The brain would be instructing the rest of the body to do whatever it takes to maintain that original body weight set point, such as slow down calorie expenditure.

Researchers have examined the brain's role in weight management, particularly in relation to hunger and satiety. One highly cited 2007 study suggested that since the hippocampus contains many leptin and insulin receptors, it could play a crucial role in appetite strength as a form of a memory or learned behavior. [17] Researchers also stated that people with a history of energy dysregulation, such as obesity, could be particularly sensitive to these hippocampal satiety signals. Further, if the hippocampus is damaged, such as in a person with amnesia, this could interfere with the satiety signal, causing the person to overeat. Theoretically, the hippocampus, which is involved in memory, inhibits people's intake of food because they remember having eaten already. The brain and hormones thus play a powerful role governing appetite and weight management.

Key Takeaway 8

Obesity has multiple causes and therefore requires several different targets and treatments to overcome each individual factor.

Analysis

To target the wide range of factors that cause obesity, such as sugar, carbohydrates, and insulin resistance, an individual must take an approach that targets each factor. Any aspect of a diet that lowers the fat storage hormone insulin can be effective. General guidelines include reducing consumption of added sugars and refined grains, moderating protein consumption, and increasing consumption of natural fats and protective factors, such as fiber and vinegar.

These general guidelines, while meant to preclude following any particular diet, do align with a diet that has surfaced in the past year: the "pegan" diet. The pegan diet combines aspects of the Paleo and vegan diets and has been popularized by Mark Hyman. [18] Pegan dieters avoid sugar and refined carbohydrates, and choose foods that are low in or devoid of pesticides, antibiotics, and hormones. The pegan diet is high in vegetables, fruit, and healthy fats, and includes adequate protein intake. These factors align the pegan diet with general dietary guidelines for combating obesity through the reduction of high levels of insulin and insulin resistance.

Author's Style

As a physician, Jason Fung relies heavily on scientific studies to explain his viewpoints on obesity and disprove common myths and problematic assumptions. Many of these studies are from the past decade, but some date back several decades to show the progression of nutrition and obesity research over time. Fung makes a point to focus on causal factors instead of association studies because associations aren't as concrete or helpful as causation. Alongside scientific research, he describes biological processes that depict how different systems of the body work together to cause either weight gain and obesity or weight loss.

Fung outlines what obesity is and how it came to be such a major societal problem. He then deconstructs the myths that surround it. He uses a biological model to explain the gradual onset of obesity and the biological and environmental factors involved. He then discusses the social phenomena associated with obesity, the problems inherent in the standard Western diet, and finally the solution to obesity, namely what to eat and when to eat it. He includes appendices that provide meal plans and practical guides to fasting, stress reduction, and sleep hygiene, all of which aid in the implementation of effective obesity treatment.

Author's Perspective

Jason Fung is a kidney disease specialist who has gained insight into obesity by treating patients suffering from type 2 diabetes, the most common cause of kidney failure. Fung developed the Intensive Dietary Management (IDM) program, which integrates a low-carb diet with proper meal timing to treat patients with diabetes. Many IDM practitioners eventually are able to discontinue their insulin use. This is an important goal of IDM, as Fung argues that high levels of insulin and insulin resistance are two primary causes of obesity.

~~~~ END OF INSTAREAD ~~~~

Thank you for purchasing this Instaread book

**Download the Instaread mobile app to get
unlimited text & audio summaries
of bestselling books.**

Visit Instaread.co
to learn more.

References

1. The Nielsen Company. "We Are What We Eat: Healthy Eating Trends Around the World." The Nielsen Company, January 2015. Accessed April 8, 2016. http://www.nielsen.com/content/dam/nielsenglobal/eu/nielseninsights/pdfs/Nielsen%20Global%20Health%20and%20Wellness%20Report%20-%20January%202015.pdf

2. Thomas, Diana, and Steven B. Heymsfield. "Exercise: Is More Always Better?" *Current Biology* 26.3 (2016): R102-R104. Accessed April 8, 2016. http://www.cell.com/current-biology/abstract/S0960-9822(15)01557-2

3. Pontzer, Herman, et al. "Constrained Total Energy Expenditure and Metabolic Adaptation to Physical Activity in Adult Humans." *Current Biology* 26.3 (2016): 410-417. Accessed April 25, 2016. http://www.cell.com/current-biology/abstract/S0960-9822(15)01577-8

4. Mohamed, Waleed S. "Role of Ghrelin, Leptin and Insulin Resistance in Development of Metabolic Syndrome in Obese Patients." *Endocrinology & Metabolic Syndrome* 3:122. January 30, 2014. Accessed April 25, 2016. http://www.omicsonline.org/open-access/role-of-ghrelin-leptin-and-insulin-resistance-in-development-of-metabolic-syndrome-in-obese-patients-2161-1017.1000122.php?aid=22700

5. Schwarz, Neil A., et al. "A Review of Weight Control Strategies and Their Effects on the Regulation of Hormonal Balance." *Journal of Nutrition and Metabolism* 2011 (2011): 15 pgs. Accessed April 25, 2016. http://www.hindawi.com/journals/jnme/2011/237932/

6. Guldbrand, H., et al. "In type 2 diabetes, randomisation to advice to follow a low-carbohydrate diet transiently improves glycaemic control compared with advice to follow a low-fat diet producing a similar weight loss." *Diabetologia* 55 (2012): 2118-2127. Accessed April 8, 2016. http://link.springer.com/article/10.1007%2Fs00125-012-2567-4

7. The Nielsen Company.

8. Strom, Stephanie. "Cereals Begin to Lose Their Snap, Crackle and Pop." *The New York Times,* September 10, 2014. Accessed April 8, 2016. http://www.nytimes.com/2014/09/11/business/cereals-struggle-in-us-as-tastes-and-rituals-change.html?_r=0

9. World Health Organization. "WHO calls on countries to reduce sugars intake among adults and children." March 4, 2015. Accessed April 8, 2016. http://www.who.int/mediacentre/news/releases/2015/sugar-guideline/en/

10. US Food and Drug Administration. "FDA revises proposed Nutrition Facts label rule to

include a daily value for added sugars." July 24, 2015. Accessed April 8, 2016. http://www.fda.gov/NewsEvents/Newsroom/PressAnnouncements/ucm455837.htm

11. Falbe, Jennifer, et al. "Higher Retail Prices of Sugar-Sweetened Beverages 3 Months After Implementation of an Excise Tax in Berkeley, California." *American Journal of Public Health* 105.11 (2015): 2194-2201. Accessed April 8, 2016. http://ajph.aphapublications.org/doi/abs/10.2105/AJPH.2015.302881

12. Evich, Helena Bottemiller. "War over soda taxes coming to a polling place near you." *Politico*, November 29, 2015. Accessed April 8, 2016. http://www.politico.com/story/2015/11/war-over-soda-taxes-coming-to-a-polling-place-near-you-216216

13. Yang, Qing. "Gain weight by 'going diet?' Artificial sweeteners and the neurobiology of sugar cravings." *Yale Journal of Biology and Medicine* 83.2 (2010): 101-108. Accessed April 8, 2016. http://www.ncbi.nlm.nih.gov/pmc/articles/PMC2892765/

14. An, Ruopeng. "Beverage Consumption in Relation to Discretionary Food Intake and Diet Quality among US Adults, 2003 to 2012." *Journal of the Academy of Nutrition and Dietetics* 116.1 (2016): 28-37. Accessed April

8, 2016. http://www.andjrnl.org/article/
S2212-2672(15)01258-7/abstract

15. Palmer, Sharon. "Nutritional Anomaly – Might
Antinutrients Offer Some Benefits?" *Today's
Dietitian* 13.7 (2011): 54. Accessed April 8,
2016. http://www.todaysdietitian.com/newar-
chives/070111p54.shtml

16. Slavin, Joanne. "Fiber and Prebiotics:
Mechanisms and Health Benefits." *Nutrients*
5.4 (2013): 1417-1435. Accessed April 8, 2016.
http://www.ncbi.nlm.nih.gov/pmc/articles/
PMC3705355/

17. Davidson, T.L., et al. "A Potential Role for
the Hippocampus in Energy Intake and
Body Weight Regulation." *Current Opinion in
Pharmacology* 7, 6 (2007): 613-616. Accessed
April 8, 2016. http://www.ncbi.nlm.nih.gov/
pmc/articles/PMC2223183/

18. Hyman, Mark. "Why I am a Pegan – or
Paleo-Vegan – and Why You Should Be Too!"
Dr. Mark Hyman. Updated April 6, 2016.
Accessed April 8, 2016. http://drhyman.com/
blog/2014/11/07/pegan-paleo-vegan/

Lightning Source UK Ltd.
Milton Keynes UK
UKOW06f1600140617
303283UK00027B/500/P